Platform Papers

Quarterly essays from Currency House

No. 4: April 2005

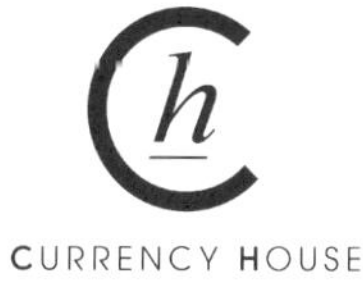

PLATFORM PAPERS

Quarterly essays from Currency House Inc.

Editor: Dr John Golder, j.golder@unsw.edu.au

Currency House Inc. is a non-profit association and resource centre advocating the role of the performing arts in public life by research, debate and publication.

Postal address: PO Box 2270, Strawberry Hills, NSW 2012, Australia

Email: info@currencyhouse.org.au Tel: (02) 9319 4953

Website: www.currencyhouse.org.au Fax: (02) 9319 3649

ISBN 0 9757301 0 X

ISSN 1449-583X

National Library of Australia Cataloguing-in-publication Data

Archer, Robyn, 1948– .

The myth of the mainstream: politics and performing arts in Australia today.

ISBN 0 9757301 0 X.

1. Arts and society – Australia. 2. Performing arts – Australia. 3. Australia – Cultural policy. I. Title. (Series: Platform papers; no. 4).

790.20994

Cover design by Kate Florance

Typeset in 10.5 Arrus BT

Printed by Hyde Park Press, Adelaide

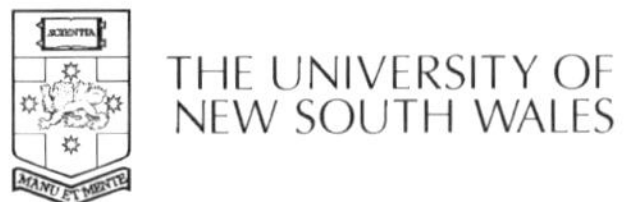

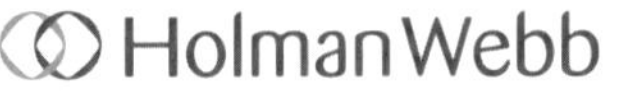

The publication of *Platform Papers* is assisted by the University of New South Wales, Holman Webb Lawyers (Australia) and Gleebooks.

Contents

AVAILABILITY *Platform Papers*, quarterly essays on the performing arts, is published every January, April, July and October and is available through bookshops or by subscription (for order form, see page 72).

LETTERS Currency House invites readers to submit letters of 400–1,000 words in response to the essays. Letters should be emailed to the Editor at j.golder@unsw.edu.au or posted to Currency House at PO Box 2270, Strawberry Hills, NSW 2012, Australia. To be considered for the next issue, the letters must be received by 4 May 2005.

CURRENCY HOUSE For membership details, see our website at: www.currencyhouse.org.au

The Myth of the Mainstream

Politics and the performing arts in Australia today

ROBYN ARCHER

Author's acknowledgements

Like most things in the last frenetic thirty years of my life, this essay has demanded working on the run, with little time for consultation. I want to acknowledge all those friends and colleagues in Australia and around the world for their generous and challenging conversations in after-show theatres and bars, in dressing-rooms, formal forums, offices, cars and cafés. Long may they continue, and forever may we remain curious!

Thanks in particular to David Young, with whom I was able to grab one couch conversation on this topic between our respective international flights, to Katharine Brisbane for her courage and wisdom, and to John Golder for his patient and careful editing.

Nothing I have done, or do, would have been possible in quite the same way without the continuing influence of my late mentor John Willett.

The author

Robyn Archer, AO, is a singer, writer and director. Having performed in recent years in Zurich, Berlin, New York and Oxford, as well as Australia, she is currently preparing a new work with Paul Grabowsky and the Australian Art Orchestra. After ten years in London, where her one-woman show, *A Star is Torn*, ran for a year in the West End, Robyn returned to Australia, where she has developed new dimensions to her career: she has been the Chair of the Australia Council's Community Cultural Board and was Artistic Director of the National Festival of Australian Theatre (1993–95), the Adelaide Festival (1998–2000), the Melbourne International Festival of Arts (2002–04) and created a new festival for Tasmania, Ten Days on the Island, with which she has been associated since its inauguration in 2001. She is currently Artistic Director of Liverpool, European Capital of Culture, 2008 and continues to serve on a number of arts-related boards in Australia. Robyn is a Chevalier de l'ordre des arts et des lettres (France), and been given honorary doctorates by Flinders (SA) and Sydney Universities.

Introduction

The main thrust of this essay is a lament for the loss of dialectic in our society. It is not a yearning for the past or a whinge about the present. There are fertile young minds ready to take on the challenges of the future and many offer an optimistic world view. It's hard to imagine that art will not have a place in that future, and the kind of art it should be is always up for discussion in any era. Unfortunately, the kind of art that wants to occupy a central place in society currently lacks a strong Australian backer. It is not respected and is accordingly undervalued and under-resourced. Occupied by debate, discussion, informed and knowledgeable analysis of past and present, intellectual, moral and ethical rigour, the transient space that dialectic occupies is a place where life's state of flux and contraries are on show. It is a place that is also occupied by art and artists. If that space is nullified or discredited—or, in some repressive societies, banned altogether—then art that wants to matter struggles to exist. I am suggesting that space is threatened, that dialectic has been usurped by dogma, that fixed opinion for opinion's sake has replaced the individual's ability to reason, and that this condition of national life has the tendency to stifle the essence of art.

The re-election of a Howard government for a fourth term,[1] and the platform which served both Labor and the Coalition in the pre-election campaign, tell me that many people in Australia today have bought the idea of a 'mainstream'. I can't say a 'majority' of Australians believe there is a homogeneous mainstream, because the fact is our governments are never elected by simple majorities. But I do think we have witnessed the fabrication of a myth which many people have bought. Belief in this myth presents a potential threat both to many people in our society and to some outside our country, because the myth of a mainstream also encourages fantasies about those who are *not* part of the mainstream.

The word 'minority' is not just descriptive: it diminishes the social status of its subject, whereas the mainstream myth might be debunked by the revelation of just how much common ground exists between the so-called mainstream and those currently portrayed as clinging to the banks or swimming against the tide. But the 2004 federal election did not debate those issues of common ground, and rarely elevated itself to questions of morals, ethics or humanity. It focused on greed and those things which reinforce the myth of the mainstream. It is part of the myth that matters of health and wages are unquestionably about 'mainstream' values. The fact is that those debates were already conducted within the discourse of a mythical mainstream. For a start, much of the economic debate only concerned the garnering of votes and, given the increase in the vote-sensitive numbers of an ageing population, it was no surprise to find hips and teeth on the national agenda: we heard little about Aboriginal health, and at no time was there, nor is there now, any attempt to align money spent on health with the money gained by government through tobacco, gambling and alcohol taxes. There was a thinly disguised desperation shown for an increase in white Australian numbers through more baby money, but little attempt to contextualise how, for instance, the urgent environmental challenges which are not currently being met will affect the life and health of those new babies.

The other side of this same coin ensures that human beings outside this alleged mainstream, no matter how populous they might be in their own countries, are granted minority status in the minds of many Australians—just as they are if they find themselves caught in the unpleasant, sometimes horrific, quest for political asylum on these shores. Regarding other human beings as 'minor', or not quite as human as 'we' are, is a time-dishonoured method of giving the 'mainstream' permission to persecute and discriminate at home, or declare war on them abroad. It is a process of brutalisation.

In the absence of dialectic, or even simple debate, there are few means whereby the public can be urged to question who exactly constitutes this mainstream. My belief is that if people were encouraged to scratch the surface of those lives politically marketed to be seen to share so many important values, they would find significant differences in the detail of their opinions, and deeper down, in the skeletons in their closet, surprising tastes, their intellectual flexibility, their real financial picture and so much more. This is the public to whom, in curating festivals, I refuse to condescend. When asked by my marketing manager, 'Who is this show for?', my reply is always, 'Whomever you can attract to it. It's for anyone who can be persuaded to attend.' I don't like reductive marketing. Somewhere there will be a kid from a battling family, a kid who sees something new and unexpected, and for whom that something will resound for the rest of her life. In many places there will be people like those in branches of my own family, on welfare, not well-educated, with kids who have problems, and whose aspirations are much more like those of my parents. They do their best and just hope their kids survive. They have no room for much vision beyond that, but are nevertheless ready and willing to respond to unusual and new works of art with a refreshing energy and direct commentary not obfuscated by artspeak. Yet one aspect of the myth is that the mainstream is scared of art.

This kind of wild suburban rumour plays into the hands of conservative power. Contact with art can sometimes have an effect that results in change or challenge. It is not necessarily always art with a message that does this. Contact with sheer beauty can often do it. It may very well send a strongly affected audience member careering off the path of so-called mainstream values on a hunt for the individual self. This is sometimes decried as selfishness. The Australian thing to do is not to be selfish, not to rock the boat too much, and the Australian people are saying broadly, 'Let's keep things nice, the way they are.' The truth of the matter is that a lot of 'the Australian thing' is very nice indeed. We have a warm and picturesque landscape, genuinely exciting modern cities; and the country abounds in stories of human kindness, community projects and volunteer service. But we also have a disenfranchised Indigenous population, an exodus of brainpower, a shameful record on refugees and, for the first time in our history, we have recently made war on a country which did not attack us. The anomaly is that, while volunteer service to clubs or to sport is much praised, those who want to visit kids incarcerated in the Baxter Detention Centre are regarded as troublemakers.

Walls of any kind, those with real barbed wire and those that block out heart and vision, are symptomatic of a society fearful that it will lose what it has. The more the mainstream want to keep it the way it is, the higher the wall they have to build to keep change out. But we know from history that it never stays that way, and the higher the wall, the bigger the inevitable crash. Of course, that sometimes doesn't happen in our own lifetime—so who is selfish now? In political life it's often a matter of 'as long as it doesn't happen in my term of office'—the ultimate selfishness.

What drives all of this, as many have already noted, is fear. Stay in your own place, align with each other, draw to the middle of the road, and ensure that the enemy is named, even when all sorts of enemies today are nameless and faceless. I counterpoint this with the idea of courage, epitomised in the kind of art in which people have the courage to do what they most believe in and to stand up in public and allow their lives to be examined in detail through their work. As a redoubtable and exceedingly wise ex-ABC journalist said to me in Melbourne last October, 'Old age is not for wimps.' That seems to be true, and I would add that art is not for wimps either.

Marketing the myth of the mainstream has been a convenient way to back people into association through the lowest common denominator, and while they're fenced in they can be branded—for us or agin us. The word 'mainstream' has taken on pernicious and equally mythical attributes such as 'Australian', so that being 'outside the mainstream' is seen as being 'un-Australian'. Yet all the time we could have aimed for the stars and set difference and complexity as the hallmarks of a great twenty-first-century society. We might have insisted that the highest common denominator be used to determine the way we associate, rather than the lowest, which are perennially set to divide us: income, education, retirement and law enforcement are all states of inevitable inequality in the late capitalist state.

And while entertainment flourishes in the superficial, smoothed-over public domain, the conditions required for art are quite different. We need the careful tendering of the complex points of difference and the maintaining of interest in subtle places between the cracks in society. These are the spaces where art is made … and right now it's a tough time for art.

1
Two days in Tasmania

Saturday 20 November 2004, Hobart—evening of the Christmas Pageant Day

I read with a kind of calm horror Frank Devine's column in yesterday's *Australian*. It was the day for 'Arts on Friday', a week or two after the launch of the Sydney and Perth Festivals and the day after the launch of Ten Days on the Island.[2] Two pages (except for the adverts) were devoted to the arts and three-quarters of one to the new Museum of Modern Art in New York. As always, I don't resent reading about MOMA—I'll be there soon to see it. What bothers me is the fact that the hundreds of rich stories about the artists creating work for those three festivals will never be told in the national daily.

Meanwhile Frank Devine's prose wears a hideous smirk. 'It's our turn,' the smile of power says. He demeans a huge number of Australians as the 'deconstructionist left' and, most misleadingly, states that their political antecedents only date back to the 1960s. He revels in the fact that the country is in a conservative mood and that abortion can again be debated, when even the Prime Minister is having to state and state again that it is a woman's right to choose. I start wondering whether the current American

First Lady and her daughters exert influence beyond the President to the Australian Prime Minister. I agree that the debate on abortion, like all debates, might be worth having again, but not when it is no debate at all, just a thinly veiled return to repression. I shudder at Devine's triumphalism. It brings closer to reality the irrational thought that one day certain Australians, some artists for instance, might have to suffer for their beliefs. Persecution now seems all too possible.

Because Frank's right about the way people voted. Despite the continuing anomaly of every state having a Labor government, enough people in Australia as a whole have decided again, and convincingly, that they feel safer with a conservative federal government. (The same applies, by and large, to the USA, of course.[3]) It is so convincing that there are only two ways to go for those who still see things they want to change—they can crawl back into covert dissent and disappointment, or else their thought and work can become re-energised and more overtly political.

Sunday 21 November 2004, Hobart

I watch the final of *Australian Idol 2*. Casey Donovan is a big girl at sixteen.[4] She has sung off-pitch every time I've heard her. Anthony Callea is tiny and good looking and has a fine, straight voice. He sings on pitch. Search me, but he looks more marketable than Casey. It's not just winners and losers, they remind us—they show the others, those who didn't get through but are carving out careers all the same. I can't knock it. I did the same thing when I was 16; it was called *Bandstand*

Starflight International. I made the national final in my second-to-last year at high school, and the next year Helen Reddy won it. It was important to me. For someone from a family without resources this was an opportunity. For a farmed-out Dad who took on tent-boxing, or a petite Piaf reaching from the gutter to the stars, it's always been that way—boxing for boys, singing for girls. Filled with the fear of shame, I had seen Dad trying out in the early talent quests when TV first came in—*Stairway to the Stars*. Mum and I watched in fear for his humiliation. He wasn't made for TV.

All the same, as they draw out the final announcement, live over-enthusiasm betrays the real intent—'Anytime now, and there can only be one winner.' Right. I can't help but see the manipulation. Judges Mark Holden and Ian ('Dicko') Dickinson are also moulded as personalities—their human faces are all to the fore. We are not told the detail of the financial arrangements made for the kids, who have to sign up to their management and recording contracts respectively. Not that anyone is covering this up. It's all known, if not understood. Welcome to twenty-first-century Australia, where, as long as you've heard it on the news and talked about it at dinner, you have no more responsibility—no further action required. Marcia Hines, the third judge, most likely doesn't have a nasty bone in her body in any case, but, because this is the vehicle which has re-launched her singing career, she must be seen to be nice to everyone. It is all feel-good spectacle and when I hear Anthony sing I warm to him, because he has a good voice and he dares to sing in Italian. I know he won't win. The suburbs are voting. The voters are mainly girls and we already know that girls don't vote for rival females; as for the boys, while they'll go for the 'fro, they won't quite get a grip on Anthony's height.

Casey is a battler. She's young and overweight and comes from Bankstown. There are lots of girls out there like her, who sympathise with her, and who've just *sms*ed the producers and Telstra a small fortune. It has something to do with Casey's talent—she's OK, she has heart, and she'll learn to sing better, she'll acquire pitch—but much more with the sociology of the voters. And are the producers looking to her studies, to her future? (We see she's already been awfully humiliated by a mistake writ large in the public media: they got the website address wrong and kids were logging on to another Casey Donovan, a US male porn star.) She's young. If she can't keep this up she'll come an awful cropper, because then she'll have been given 'the big chance' and she'll end up still overweight and now a failure. I hope they're taking care of the downside, though somehow I doubt it. I am inclined to enjoy the moment, but I don't see very much original about Casey's voice and, unlike Anthony's, it seems at the edge of her capability. Big girls Mama Cass and Alison Moyet had better voices and their weight got in the way of sustained success. But this is not about history or reason, and not about a sustained career. This is about commerce and tribalism, the marks of that mainstream to which we are meant to aspire.

I switch channels to *Compass*, which is about Guy Sebastian's Church in Paradise, South Australia.[5] I know Paradise. In my time it was a much-maligned locality and there were always jokes about the buses being 'bound for Paradise'. I learn that the church is Pentecostal and that they tolerate neither divorce, nor sex before marriage, nor homosexuals. This sweet, angel-voiced boy whom the nation voted for last year disapproves of, perhaps condemns, me for my choice of partners, and condemns many of my dearest friends because they chose abortion. But it's not just the Pentecostals. The Coalition and the Labor Party have also forbidden same-sex marriage. I think of all those couples who have fought so hard for recognition within their own extended families—now subject again to discrimination and lack of respect. Their love is outside the law, outside the mainstream and legislated against. And the anti-abortion league is on the rise again. Frank Devine rejoices in all this. It would be easy for many to resign themselves to a despised fate.

Rebelling against post-war calm, challenging the subservient lives many saw their mothers live, challenging a government that sent many a brother to fight and die in another country's unjust war, we were encouraged to live lives truer to ourselves and to elevate the role that creativity plays in a healthy society. Now the cycle has finally moved into its next phase and we must hope that the creativity which drove our finest hopes will drive us again to bring about a return to somewhere that is not running scared, not destructively competitive, that is humane rather than tribal and that is proud of its artists as well as its entertainers. I think of the phenomenal economic success of Iceland and that an Icelandic parent's proudest experience is seeing their offspring become a poet.

2
Aspiring to what?

There is still more of the artist than the cultural commentator in me, and my materials are those of my life, so I crave your indulgence and ask you to forgive the personal. Was I spawned in a mainstream? Certainly, I was bred of two battlers and, in a post-war moment when, believing one to be quite enough, they would have spurned Treasurer Peter Costello's recent call to legover.[6] Their tastes were for entertainment not art, as were mine. Cliff was a stand-up comic, MC and self-taught singer. Mary played piano 'by ear'. They loved a good sing. I don't believe they would ever have bought a ticket to a performance: it would always have been, and still is, thought beyond their fragile pocket. The 'pictures', as they were called, were our special entertainment. Still, if I provided them with tickets to see art, they always enjoyed it and always spoke intelligently of even the weirdest stuff. That has remained a touchstone for me.

What were the aspirations of this couple? Cliff would have loved to go on being a professional entertainer full-time, but now he had a wife and kid and so he needed a stable income. It was never stable: the pub work for Charlie, who let him down in the end and didn't leave him the pub when he retired; the car-yard mechanic's job, which folded in the '61 credit squeeze, when Cliff had to go truck-driving to Mount

Isa and Mary and I cried for weeks. All Mary wanted was a home of her own—which she never got. What she did get was an ex-gambler, afraid to get a mortgage because he couldn't bear being in debt again, and a child so ill with asthma that she feared, as the doctors said, that she might never raise her. What they wanted for this kid was 'health and happiness', as Mary always signed her letters to me when I lived in London. I'm not sure that the idea of 'mainstream' existed then: there were rich and poor, a middle class and battlers like us. There were no marketing campaigns as such around elections and no appeals to aspirational Australians. But then, both parties favoured cheap, rented housing for those who could not afford to buy, free education and free health services.

In the most recent federal election, was the word 'aspirational' not shorthand for 'I aspire to have more money'? Of course, most people want to have good health care and good education services, good garbage collection, an honest police force, and decent food and shelter. But 'aspirational'? Unfortunately, the ideal of capitalism has been in some ways as disappointing in practice as the ideal of communism. Capitalism has not ensured an everyone's-a-winner society. If it had, hit TV shows like *Who Wants to be a Millionaire?* would not be hits. Capitalism as we know it relies on a have- and a have-not society. Sadly, 'winners' also implies 'losers'. 'Aspirational' has the smack of winners and losers—if you aspire to a better lifestyle and you work for it, then you may get it—but one thing is for sure, not everyone will get it, often those who most aspire to it. There will be some very sore losers.

And what of those Australians who do aspire to be poets, who aspire to dance, or write, or play music, for their living? Some say there will now be a period of attrition, not altogether undesirable. Some talk about a new breed of very savvy artists who can already be seen today. They have jobs in some commercial application of their art (design or media). On the side they have a collective that gets a café together—coffee, exhibition space, club, live music and performance space. It's cool, it's hip, and it's popular. They scrape together support in kind through friends and connections. They are savvy. But is the art everything we want from art, or does the necessity for cool mean that this stuff is governed by fashion? Will it rock the boat and floor the soul, or will it play into the pleasant groove of a tidy city life?

But isn't that OK? Surely, those involved have their own benchmarks of complexity and wit: it is not possible to claim simply that one age is smarter than another. The main problem with work that follows fashion is that it might not have the energy to stir people into action—and if there is no action, then some will live in a very pleasant place, but injustices will continue to occur and not all the world will choose to turn a blind eye to them. The place within itself may be a paradise for some—but it may lose its ethical standing in the world, as Australia already has in many parts of Asia and Europe.

A lot of what Chris Latham says in *Survival of the Fittest*,[7] and what composer David Young too has discussed in conversation with me about the future of the collective, is reflected from the other side by Paul

Carter, who refuses to generalise about the process of art and wants not to talk in the kind of superficialities that sound-byte culture demands.[8] Carter has started to resist the quick overview (the most appropriate form for event mentality) of works which cannot be communicated easily in a few sentences, and which naturally resist perfect packaging. He writes in tiny, infinitesimal detail, with no fat, about the facts of the way in which art is produced. In some ways this practical recording of process from the viewpoint of the rigorous and articulate academic/practitioner is worlds apart from the savvy café/gallery model, but in many ways it says the same thing—that the way you put work together is fragmented, not easy, and in the end collaborative, with genuine give-and-take, learning and re-learning.

Is there still space in this world for the individual who is not at the top of the hierarchy? What, indeed, of the weirdo who simply wants to pursue the work, outside of the mainstream of fashion? Will it mean that such an artist is again destined for a lifetime of neglect, with the possibility of being re-discovered in a hundred years' time? Many enduring artists never knew fame or comfort while they were alive. Being an artist is not for wimps. Is it just the way of the world that, if you want people to look at your art and you want to earn money from it, you have no choice but to be savvy about it and hope you can ride the line between earning a quid and not losing sight of what your art set out to do in the first place? It is the Kafka decision: 'My art will never feed me. I have to have a job and will make my art in my spare time.'

This will be part of the attrition, and in accord with history. A number of enduring artists have taken this course.

This was my own dilemma in Sydney in the early '70s. Earning well from the clubs for three days' work should have given me time to practise the things I really wanted. But it didn't work. I spent the whole time being so worried about the medium where I wasn't a good fit that I had neither the time nor energy to spend on the work I really wanted to pursue. What was the nature of that clubland compromise that I couldn't hack?

I had just been through four years at university in an intensive English Language and Literature course that went from translating *Beowulf* and the Early English Mystics, through Shakespeare, then Milton, Dryden and Blake, then Gibbon, Richardson and Smollett, into James, Eliot and Lawrence, and at last contemporary—even our own—creative writing. I was forced to absorb critics like Leavis and Empson and, long before I had the mental capacity or world experience to do so, adopt a critical stance of my own. But the main thing I was absorbing was the ability to go deeper, to look for infinite subtlety and cross reference. What the clubs wanted, what the audience wanted—and what many artists were perfectly prepared, happy and fulfilled to give them—was whatever was popular. It was not subtle, it had no depth, it was what people already knew and wanted. You gave it to them, or you didn't get booked—it was as straightforward as that. I resisted by working a creatively structured repertoire of lesser-known works in the mould, and it sort of worked. The ultimate realisation, however, was that there were entertainers who really enjoyed this. I came to see that I didn't. I aspired to something more.

It is the absence of subtlety and intellectual rigour that I fear most at present. There is a priest, a long-time supporter of the arts, who works in the suburbs of Melbourne. Having had to defend his faith vigorously during the heady 1960s, he says now that he's appalled by young people in his parish who come to him saying, 'I don't want to question or debate, just give me the dogma and I'll obey.' This fits the brief of the mainstream fiction currently maintained by both our major parties: we are a nation of ordinary, good people and we will provide mainly for things that ordinary, good people want. We are a simple, open, outdoor, sport-loving, fun-loving nation. It is enough for us simply to be ourselves; we do not need to 'improve' ourselves. We do not wish to debate the hard issues. We only want to know we have enough cash with which to live well and see our kids live well. And we are happy with politicians who tell us that these are their concerns too. Australia is a world of ordinary people, happy to gossip on talk-back radio, but not to value the structures and resources (including art) that allow us to develop our critical and analytical powers. It makes us seem more and more like the America we see on daytime interview shows and have long criticised. But at least the candidates in last year's American presidential campaign were required to debate on policy. We didn't get that, we got sniping. There was a moment when a group of eminent minds gathered together to make a public criticism of government policy. They were howled down as opposition stooges and irrelevant academics. A climate of this sort is not one to breed artists who will dig into the depths, who have the potential to inspire and awaken the hidden richness in us all. Superficiality and public deception do not provide fertile ground in which art can take root and grow.

A prejudice against the intellectual, a preference for pure entertainment, the lack of training and practice in following things through to a logical conclusion and the refusal to examine consequences, the adherence to 'in or out', 'black or white'—these are some of the consequences of falling for the myth of the mainstream, while all along in their own families this so-called mainstream is allowing for difference, tolerating compromise, allowing a son or daughter to talk them round on an issue of race or sex or music or exploitation. But in public the beast of the mainstream denies these quiet acts of deliberation and change—and that's its danger—especially for the arts, where most of the changes they effect are not monumental, but quietly and seepingly subversive.

3
The death of dialectic

When I wrote the feisty political songs of my youth, there was no doubt in my mind that one blamed the country's leader for the ills of the nation. It was hard when I began to think that perhaps it is true that a country gets the government it deserves—and even now I'm not sure that, given their diverse histories, that is true for all countries. But one thing I am sure of in Australia today is that a leader cannot be held wholly and solely responsible for failure to take action on all the things I would like to see changed. Understandably, all politicians have one vital thing in mind, to remain popular enough to be re-elected. If re-elected, they then pursue policies which they believe, many truly in their hearts, are best for the country. But for only a short while do anxieties about re-election subside, allowing time for genuine policy-making. There are very few brave enough to go against the tide of popular opinion. Even those who appear to be making a brave stand are more likely to be voicing the accepted position of their supporters: it may not be a widely-held position, but enough to satisfy the numerical minority who have been targeted. In a market driven world, a successful politician knows his market and delivers it the goods.

When a government is as decisively elected for a fourth term, electoral boundaries and preferential voting systems notwithstanding, we have to acknowledge that enough people (around half in John Howard's case) believe that what those politicians have been doing in the last three terms is acceptable, even praiseworthy. It's likely that many are either turning a blind eye to political convenience, or have simply lost the ability to reason things to their logical conclusion. Where monochrome opinion dominates, where changing your mind or wavering is considered a weakness rather than a noble attribute, there is little room for real questions and real debate.

During his 2004 Melbourne International Arts Festival performance, *The Charcoal Club—for Singed Whites and Burnt-out Blacks*, Richard J. Frankland showed edited clips of his interview with Germaine Greer. Many simply found it laughable. The tendency to ridicule the perennially interesting and headline-grapping prof. has most recently manifested itself on the occasion of her entrance into the house of the UK's *Celebrity Big Brother*—and exit, pursued by the octogenarian Jackie Stallone. While I applaud Dr Greer's actions here, I had real issues with the speech she made in London in December 2003: she pilloried a well-known Aboriginal artist who was unknown to most of her English audience, but gave him no right of reply. On the other hand I don't entirely dismiss her claim that the only way for Australia to move forward is to become an Aboriginal nation. I think it's wholly impractical and will never, in my opinion, happen, but I do think we need the space to dream and to take the time to think things through, instead of immediately taking up combative positions. For me, that attitude of being with'em or agin'em, being a winner or a loser, being 'in or out'—*Australian Idol* is by no means the only popular cultural manifestation of this; there's *Big Brother, Who Wants to be a Millionaire?, Who's Best- and Worst-dressed?*, the ascendancy of sport as tribal spectacle rather than a forum for exercise and personal best, *My Restaurant Rules, The Great Race, Survivor*, too—this is the scariest thing about the philosophical framework within which people view life at present.

I am content to speculate on what Germaine Greer's Indigenous Republic might be like, to think about the spiritual possibilities and the practical impossibilities. It is the kind of exercise that stimulates the mind, the conscience, the ethical and creative muscles, and it provokes rigorous debate, too. It's a good thing to do—but it's very unpopular. For any political leader today even to contemplate publicly such a scenario would invite accusations of irresponsibility, and almost certainly guarantee electoral defeat. Yet such an exercise lies at the core of why we are human and, apparently, the most advanced species on the planet.

Following the widespread discrediting of Stalinism and the gradual collapse of various Communist states, most of what Marx wrote has been dismissed. The fact that young people, especially in Eastern Europe, are turning to his writings again should alert us to the thought that a good deal of what he said might be worth preservation. There was a time when Communism was the hope of nations, a new kind of internationalism that would unite the world in compassion and co-operation, not unlike the spirit of many current worldwide movements.

One of the greatest losses is the neglect of the process of dialectic, in which we pitch theory against theory, counter one opinion with another, in order to reason the most logical and truthful conclusion *at that time*. Inherent in the theory of dialectic is the idea that there is no absolute truth and that sooner or later currently held truths will be overturned. One reason for the failure of Communism in practice was precisely the inability to acknowledge transience—the mistake of setting in concrete a new society which itself would one day need to be overturned. I also observe that it is fear of transience, a condition in which nothing is sure for ever, that drives people to avoid thinking too clearly and to opt for tribal safety (which being in the mainstream is) and romanticised ideas of immortality and eternity.

The absence of this desire and ability to look at many sides, to exercise our analytical powers and flex the ethical muscle, has many consequences for art. I don't believe in ex-cathedra pronouncements on art. Art is relative to the observer, and always coloured by context. As such, the way we value or judge art can only ever be part of a continuum that embraces many aspects of society as well as principles of art: the proof of this is in the way that works are often neglected for many years and then come into favour again. All opinion is justifiable, but only if the owner is prepared to give us the value system whence that opinion proceeds. The following are issues that have cropped up in various addresses I have made in recent years:

they are not about proposing a theory of Art. They are made more in that spirit which is repelled by cultural commentators who claim that they know the truth, that there is an absolute standard—arts critics, if you like, who do not feel the need to qualify their pronouncements with any statement of their knowledge, experience, qualifications, prejudice or preference.

My teachers demanded that their students cultivate objective criticism. I never bought it—not then, not now. We may comment on skill and craft (provided we possess a world of knowledge about those things) and we may make comparisons (provided we know where this art originated, both in traditional/historical/geographical terms and within the context of recent developments). Equipped with that knowledge, we may dare to claim that some works fall short of what has been and what is. But it is simply not good enough to make pronouncements based solely on personal taste. Hence some clarification, which I hope will throw light on art's place in relation to the mythical mainstream.

The preservation and interpretation of the canon

If government subsidy is intended partially to preserve the Western canon, and if the argument for the subsidy of 'major' (i.e. 'mainstream') companies is to a degree a museological one, why not approach the canon more seriously with this in mind? If we acknowledge that having the classics around is a good thing—and I believe it is—then how about a more thorough approach to the canon? Let's make sure that over a three-year period—at the very least—we see on our stages not only Shakespeare, but also Chekhov, Ibsen, Williams, Miller, Brecht, Beckett, Pinter et al. And, if these, why not our own Patrick White and Jack Davis? Let's ensure that we hear the less well-known Beethoven as well the best-liked. If we are to have opera, let's ensure that we program Monteverdi and Janacek, Adams and Stravinsky, alongside Verdi and Puccini. How about we take a more professional approach and allow Australians to experience the operatic canon in the same way that we try to make available to art-lovers and readers a catholic range of holdings in our galleries and libraries? Why shouldn't we regularly invite the Beijing Opera through our opera companies? Why couldn't Kabuki or Noh be part of a theatre company's season? If subsidy is there to preserve a museological resource for the community, why not treat the programming of the performing arts in a similar way? If we are to preserve Balanchine and Martha Graham, why not Trisha Brown, Bill Forsyth and Merce Cunningham, too?

In *Trapped by the Past*, the previous essay in this series, Julian Meyrick longs for an Australian theatre that acknowledges a past, present and future. So do I. It's interesting that the visual arts and independent film/screen culture in Australia have become much more politicised and energised at the very moment when a lot of theatre has lost the plot. But this is not, as some would argue, the fault of theatre per se. In Buenos Aires and Tehran, for instance, I have experienced the most extraordinary energy in new plays—nothing experimental about them at all. In either of these two cities the finest thing a young artist can do is write and stage—often in their own living rooms—a new play. These are invariably political in one way or another, and comment, often poetically, on the mood of the times. So I am not calling for an end to old forms.

If we acknowledge the value of the canon, in all its forms, as a benchmark for interpreters, an educational grounding for the audience, a potential first contact for the young and the uninitiated, and a comforting pleasure to those familiar with them, then we must also acknowledge the value of the new and original and untested. This is the work that has no ready-made audience, precisely because that work or the artist or the form is unknown. This work is the manifestation of the creative muscle—the most important human resource of any society. And the stimulation of our creative muscle is every bit as important as—perhaps more important than—the preservation of the canon, and the resources made available for each must be at the very least equal.

I argued this in a recent address at the National Gallery of Victoria and it prompted a reaction very similar to that provoked by the idea that women should be equal with men. It started, 'But if you have all this modern work taking over…' in the way the other debate began, 'But when you have women taking over…' It's only natural that the concept of equality should pose a threat to those with the advantage—what constantly amazes me is the shameless betrayal of that fear in the public domain.

If the canon is to be preserved, and at the taxpayers' expense, then I want to see it rigorously mined for whatever new gems it may have to offer. What I don't want to see is that amazingly rich and sometimes fragile historical resource left to those with only a limited knowledge of it—and even less ability to value it—in the belief that they have done their duty to the past if they occasionally whack in a *Twelfth Night*, *Traviata* or a trad *Swan Lake*.

But at the same time as demanding that the canon be rigorously programmed, presented as energetically as possible and with a fresh approach—even when that approach is traditional, as in the case of Richard Wherrett's *Crucible*, Richard Tognetti's Mozart, or Philippe Herreweghe's Bach, for example—I would insist on the allocation of at least equal funding for new work. And with it enough funding to permit new work to be commissioned and flexible structures developed, so that fresh ideas can be grabbed and nurtured, and individual artists empowered to see their projects through. It is sad to think that for every throwaway, bums-on-seats, crowd-pleasing stocking-filler in every subscription season, four or five great little ideas or one fantastic new piece of Australian creative genius is lost. The crowd-pleaser will still be there in ten years—the great new idea may perish forever for lack of care and sustenance. What's more, it is more likely that, if properly resourced and nurtured, the great new idea will receive invitations internationally. Not that there's anything inherently wrong with the stocking filler—nothing wrong with fun and well-loved pleasures. But if it actually impedes and stifles creativity, then it is very harmful indeed, and the myth of mainstream taste will have triumphed over the reality of the real germ of art in Australia today.

The difference between art and entertainment

An entertainer sets out at best to replicate what people already know and love. The entertainer is there above all to please an audience, not to move them on. It should be no surprise that many entertainers are politically conservative. By nature they want to be loved and they don't want to rock the boat. But an artist does not set out to play to an audience. The artist makes original work that he/she has no choice but to make. The artist can only hope that the work will somewhere find an audience which responds well to the new thing which he/she has done. Many arts organisations (especially if their continuing grants depend on bums on seats), and many of the bodies which fund them, find it hard to distinguish between the two. If a programmer sets out just to please an audience, then he/she is in the business of entertainment, and this can apply to symphonic and operatic programs as readily as to more popular forms. Conversely, the most popular forms can sometimes embrace the spirit of art.

Having had a career in pure entertainment from the age of four to the age of twenty-six, I do not disparage entertainment or entertainers. It's where my great grandmother, my father and I all came from, and I frequently return to it. But I do know the difference and I would like us to acknowledge the difference, because, unless we do, we will neglect the special conditions required for the artist. If we fail to provide these conditions of growth, an enormous patch of creative flowering will wither, and that creativity is needed, not just in art but in science and engineering and environmental studies. Precisely because it also entertains and engages, art has the power to stimulate the creative muscle in people from all fields.

The resourcing of art—especially the role of government

The reason why the notion of the mainstream is important in respect of art is because it has come to dictate the terms of support for the arts. If these things work in distinct cycles—conservatism, followed by change and reform—then, like as not, official support for the arts will reflect that pattern. If the nation is falling for the myth of the mainstream, then evidence of that myth will in all likelihood be seen in the arts: people will be persuaded that a certain kind of art is 'real' art, and the art with the numbers will receive the lion's share of taxpayer dollars. We have lost the concept of enabling all, as opposed to just the bits we favour.

But the very word 'subsidy' implies a gap—between what art costs to make and maintain, and what that art can attract from an audience. The gap is covered, prior to production, in both cash and kind through commercial sponsorship, private philanthropy (from the brother to the billionaire) and government resources, whether local, state, federal or international. If there are large numbers of people who are particularly fond of a specific art form or set of artists, doesn't it follow that those people might be willing to pay for that art through the purchase of tickets and other forms of support? This is certainly the case for popular music: it has an avid audience ready to enter into a commercial transaction to get what they want.

The role of government funding should surely be to assist those arts which do not yet have the prospect of a public willing to pay—because their work is new and untried and has no audience as yet. During the 2004 Melbourne International Arts Festival, I was *In Conversation* with some terrific Belgian artists and asked how they accounted for their phenomenal output of contemporary arts. It had begun, they said, when some luminaries had decided that certain theatre companies should devote themselves exclusively to new work. Then, one courageous cultural minister took the bit between his teeth and stopped funding companies who were stuck in the rut of unimaginative tradition. Instead, he gave the money to those who would bring on new work. Now, they said, the situation needed some correction, as it had become hard to find decent classical theatre in Belgium—the canon had been neglected. Nevertheless, the initial impetus has had remarkable results.

Recently, a couple of politicians here in Australia, dealing with the arts at different levels of government, have engaged with the problem of loosening up their budgets—how to fund the innovative and the experimental, not always just by young and emerging artists, but by old farts with new ideas, too. They have heard the pleas of the so-called small-to-medium sector and want to do something about them. They may well also have become aware that many of our international successes come not through the major arts organisations, but through the smaller independent sector. There are exceptions to this: the Australian Chamber Orchestra, for example, travels very well. But festivals and seasons all over the world are now sprinkled with independent Australian artists and companies. The so-called 'major' arts organisations—as prejudicial a term as 'minority'—are the most likely custodians of the canon and are largely geared towards catering for a local audience. These politicians are sympathetic to the idea of funding part of the core costs of the operation, but then pulling back on the more commercial fare and concentrating the balance of the grant on those elements which allow for experiment.

If repertoire is inserted for no other purpose than to put bums on seats, and no attempt is made to get at something new and revealing about the work, then let the entertainment principle apply. Allow the production to be cut to the cloth that the ticket buyer will afford. We would soon find, of course, that it's the cloth many ticket buyers want: the reassuring presence of lavish sets and costumes that applies just as much to musicals as it does to opera. It's the spectacle they're after, not the substance. OK, it costs, let them pay for it. The government, by saving their contribution to this largely commercial transaction, could redistribute the savings—to the sector most desperately in need and most likely to engage with new ideas and new forms.

The most recent push to 'restructure the Australia Council' (mid-debate as I write) is telling. The principal outcome of the Nugent Report was the allocation of increased resources to the large organisations, leaving the small-to-medium and independent sector with a comparatively smaller slice of the cake.[9] While a more recent and much needed drip of $10 million to that sector is welcome, the latest bid to remove the Community Cultural Development Board and the New Media Board simply follows the same line. A conservative view of the arts still dominates and is reflected in the division of Performing Arts into the discrete sectors of Theatre, Music, Dance, Visual Arts and Opera—and this is the view that such a restructuring supports. The fact that these generic borders have disappeared in the best and most successful work all over the world means nothing to these bureaucrats—who are restructuring according to their preferred view, no matter how out of step they may be with the ways of artists in the twenty-first century. Worldwide, the most potent source of artistic vigour lies precisely in stories and practice from the community, and in the new media: these are fields in which Australian artists are leading the world. I can only hope that the Australia Council debate will produce the best thinking and that the Government will be made to see that the very rhetoric it employs about Australian values and national pride demands that greatly increased support be given to Community Cultural Development. Perhaps, by the time this essay is published, we will see CCD direct-line funded, in the same way as Opera Australia—and for the same amount. Now that would be interesting, and rather more consistent with the mainstream argument.

Robyn Archer

The detritus theory

What artists produce, the end result of what they do, is the detritus of the creative process. I suspect that entertainment differs in that respect. Here, the end result is more important because it is audience-focused. It depends on how it goes with the audience and, for anyone aiming at a particular market and relying on a successful penetration of that market, this will be so—you buy a finished product, honed for the purpose. But many artists do not have an audience in mind. In visual art, for instance, what we might buy to put on our wall is the detritus of the real act of painting, which happened in the studio. It's a helpful way of viewing art. You understand that a work is probably never finished, it is just a part of an ongoing process. But at a certain time, you abandon it—the detritus might sell. You gladly exchange it for money that can buy you the materials and time to continue with your creative process. It can certainly be so for playwrights: at a certain point you give the piece up for a production, but you will always hope for another season, rewrites, a new interpretation etc. It's a growing thing. The same goes for choreographers. While as audiences we may enjoy artistic detritus in all its forms, if we focus entirely on the product, we neglect to see just how vitally important the process is.

Seeing art in this way, even just as an exercise, means that we distinguish between the core creator—playwright, painter, composer—and the interpreter—actor, musician, director, designer, curator. Not that interpreters lack creativity: often they and the creator are one and the same. But they live in the present, they have fixed points of focus in front of an audience, and their training and daily discipline are about being prepared for that moment. Their art is transient and ephemeral. Their art is in the doing, but, no matter how many CDs they sell, the CD too is only the detritus of what they did during the live performance, whether in the studio or before an audience.

Bearing this in mind, we must never lose sight of the importance of the process and the development of art, or of the need to nurture that process in artists. This is directly relevant to the funding/resources debate: if we only fund product, if we are constantly fixated on the glossy outcomes, if all we care about are favourable reviews, then process will be neglected and the art in its turn will be impoverished. In the cut of the cake we need not only the canonical and the new, but also resources for both experiment and thinking that will not necessarily lead to an end-product. This is perhaps the most neglected area of arts funding, and I would urge that in the areas of CCD and New Media it is at the very heart of their processes and development.

The fact of change and perpetual motion

We are like flowers. We are seeded, we grow, we sprout, we blossom—and then we start to wither, and eventually we die. History, anthropology, archaeology, cosmology, biology all tell us that everything is in a constant state of flux. That which we perceive as solid is nothing but a particular concentration of particles in wild motion. Things are not always what they seem, and change is a fact of our lives. One reason why the mainstream is such a myth is that it derives from the mistaken belief that the family has continued unaltered since the 1950s. Change is viewed as damaging for the family unit, for the upbringing of kids, but change per se matters far less than how you live with change. I was grateful for a stable family unit and a mum who didn't work while I was at school, but my most vivid early memory is of my fourth year, in the dramatic and ever-entertaining British Hotel in Adelaide, which my great granddad owned and where both my parents worked. It was the changed environment that stimulated me. Aboriginal and other nomadic desert peoples have built their communities for tens of thousands of years on the basis of transience—and their kids are fine.

Perhaps facing the fact of constant change is just too fearful, even for those who pin their hopes on their kids—kids who, like certain works of art or architecture or engineering, or even thought, are seen as the passport to life beyond the grave. We don't like to think of our smallness and transience in the grand procession, so we build things around us—houses, customs, possessions, jingoism—to help distract us from the fact of change. But tsunamis and lightning, big storms and tiny microbes, all remind us of how vulnerable we are. And now modern science has provided even more elaborate schemes—kryogenic freezing of the brain, freezing of sperm and ova—to help us postpone the inevitable.

No wonder that people place highest value on those things which have survived longest, the classics. And no wonder change is so hard to take. Why are people amazed at mid-life crises? Why do they find it disturbing to want change? It's disturbing because the very things we have gone to such lengths to build and preserve will now be disrupted. And why is change frowned upon? Because change will also disturb those things which the myth of the mainstream requires in order to feed its sense of reality.

As in the micro, so in the macro. A society is intricately configured to preserve certain values, just as funding models are. Suddenly, some brave soul, an artist, perhaps, articulates the fact that things are not OK, that something's not working. Then change requires a battle rather than a debate, between those who want change and those who resist. This is a problem for art, health, urban planning, the distribution of wealth (local and global); what can't be progressed through rational debate ends up in revolution.

Where the revolutionaries get it wrong is by constructing yet another concrete edifice which in its turn will also soon need pulling down. Give me change and flexibility. Why are students turning back to the humanities and starting to spurn economics and management? It's because they've seen Dad or big sister given a redundancy package, only to discover that he or she doesn't know how to do anything else. The humanities have proven to be very adept at preparing us for flexibility in the workplace and the ability to cope with change in general.

The life-and-death importance of curiosity

When I thought back to the pre-diagnosis signs of my father's dementia, I realised that it started with the loss of curiosity. He didn't want to read the paper anymore. He lost interest in the football and the cricket. He forced himself to come to 25 shows in the 2000 Adelaide Festival I directed. Less than a year later he was diagnosed. Since then loss of curiosity has had special significance for me. I can't help thinking that once the blinkers are on, there's only one road ahead—and that leads to death. Anyone who approaches art, or virtually anything, only wishing to defend their own tastes, anyone who won't look at anything new for fear it won't be to their liking, anyone who bags something before they've seen it, might as well be dead already. They've lost their curiosity. They're winding down.

So, what to do? Try to fuel our capacity for curiosity, by venturing as much, and as far, as possible into the intellectual and aesthetic unknown. It might just put more years on our lives than any number of vitamins.

4
What place art?

What artists do is delve so much deeper beneath the habitual generalisations of public discourse. Many refuse to gloss over tiny details, but focus on them in the hope that a larger picture will emerge. This is the process of the best twentieth-century dramatists. A clutch of American playwrights are particularly adept at focusing on the minutiae of family drama, but at the same time always able to give me a vast picture of the USA: Tennessee Williams, Arthur Miller, Sam Shepard. These are paralleled by the best of their comics, Mort Sahl and the stand-up Robin Williams. It is difficult for the art of detail to be respected when the times are overwhelmed by a public taste for crude and often inaccurate generalisation.

What we find in all journalism, whether in the print or electronic media, is the cult of the ego and the all-important by-line. In this domain, opinion is all-important, strong opinion. It reminds me of living in Thatcher's Britain, where there was a similar journalistic tendency to manufacture a mainstream, disparage everything that didn't fit the myth and seek public approval for declaring war on outsiders. In that climate, many were inclined to say, 'We like her because she knows what she's doing. She's decisive, she doesn't dither'—that's it, take that, Gotcha! One of the most distressing aspects of Australian political life in recent years has been the view, becoming increasingly widespread, that taking time to deliberate is a sign of weakness. How can we live like this? A major political figure takes time to consider consequences which will affect the life and death of large numbers of people—and this is called weakness or wavering! No wonder, in this space, that there is so little tolerance for the processes of art. Give us decisive solutions! We don't care about your questions! We've dispensed altogether with dialectic, we want dogma. We don't want problems articulated, but, if they are, then make sure that it's in a 'mainstream language'! We want neat endings to our plays, the kind presented by our major companies—not that frayed, questioning exploration of the uncertain that you get in smaller independent works! We want solid and we want answers.

In this climate, the fragile questioning forms of art are not broadly appreciated, experiment is not appreciated, any mixing of forms is found unacceptable. Keep fine music where music belongs, in the recital halls and concert halls. In fact, neglect the physical and philosophical spaces urgently required for the creation and presentation of new forms which more truly reflect the realities of contemporary Australian life. Instead, let's give priority to a new drama theatre and recital hall, where forms are guaranteed to stay independent, uncontaminated and pure. While spending on new spaces for the arts is always cause for celebration, nonetheless spending of this sort is a victory for the conservative point of view—not, it must be said, that blame can be laid at the door of the Federal Government alone.

I repeat, the preservation and robust interpretation of the Western dramatic and musical canon is important for the well-being of any community, but not at the expense of new theatrical forms, new music and new mixed art forms. These are what best, and most accurately, reflect our current circumstances, and so allow us to start thinking more realistically about ourselves and our lives and human responsibilities. Art has a crucial role to play in getting us to think about our lives, but only if we allow it to play that role. And there's the danger, because it's when art escapes the strictures of being relegated to pastime that it becomes strong and vital, able to empower people to act on those things they are not happy with.

We have been living in a bread-and-circuses environment for many years now. Subtlety and detail are not appreciated. Value is placed on quantity, not quality, on sheer scale rather than pure essence. The tiny gem is unloved. Success in art—as appraised by the media and frequently by grant-givers of all kinds—is measured by box-office takings, bums on seats. Often it is on these bases alone that an annual or triennial grant will be renewed, or not. More importantly, it's hard to convince a major sponsor that your tiny gem is worth their investment. They want to know how many people you will reach. Spectacle that attracts attention also attracts support. This is why televised sport is eagerly sponsored: it reaches the vast numbers of viewers that the sponsor also wishes to reach.

There's nothing wrong with this if the state subsidises things outside the sawdust, that are too small or too unfamiliar or too subtle to attract commercial support. The dilemma we face is that currently in Australia the lion's share of arts subsidy is also going to the spectacular. This is a time-dishonoured propaganda technique, as temporarily successful in declining Rome as it was in the Third Reich. This success is being echoed as I write, in the hymns of praise for Australia's 'largest ever theatrical production'—its size and ability to pull big-spending international tourists being the main reasons why double-page spreads and prime-time TV coverage are being devoted to it. It is the Wagner *Ring* cycle, and the television story I saw last night was not about the beautiful voice and astonishing rise of Lisa Gasteen, but about the millionaire Wagner-follower from Los Angeles—and the enormous costs and monumental scale of the production.[10]

In Australian culture right now, size definitely matters. I'm glad people enjoyed the *Ring*, and particularly happy for the State Opera of South Australia, who have adventurously programmed, alongside the odd *Magic Flute* or *Bohème*, both Wagner and Louis Andriessen, and contemporary American and local works, too—in short, they have shown themselves to be the very model of a healthy, twenty-first-century opera company. But I do worry about that single greatest attractor—size.

The politics of distraction, through *Ring* cycles, Olympic or Commonwealth Games opening ceremonies, or '*Aida*s in the stadium', ensure that those arts which bring thought and responsibility back to a human scale, which strip away illusion and want to deal with life the way it really is, are not valued. And I would claim that these works are at the source of the artistic spirit. It's not that we can't enjoy the large-scale—the absolute silence of 100,000 footy fans at the Anzac Day match, or that first roar at the start of the AFL Grand Final, never fails to bring a tear to my eye, a lump to my throat, and that is the most tribal of instincts. But I want art to lift me above my primal state. I want it to fill me with awe for the human condition. I want it to expose my shortcomings, both public and private, and thereby drive me to action.

5

And criticism has failed us

Now is a highly dynamic moment for the mass media. In the face of technological and informational changes that surpass the impact of the Industrial Revolution, most are dumbed down. Hardly surprising, since tertiary education has been underfunded and the formal critical faculty desperately impaired. This is the sign of a conservative age, when citizens who articulate dissatisfaction with the status quo are regarded as a threat. In the last few years we have experienced many instances in which the public intellectual has been despised. The arts still struggle for diminishing space in the print media and coverage is relegated to lift-out lifestyle sections, rather than being placed in proximity to news and world events. Their societal worth is thus reduced and, by being grouped with entertainment, fashion and travel, they are valued in relation to the degree to which they can compete with other pastimes. The arts are not regarded, by the Australian mass print media, as among the more serious aspects of life. They are a fringe on the frock of life.

The relegation to lift-out means that next-day reviews—particularly valuable to the potential patrons of short-season and festival shows, for instance—have become a thing of the past. Reviews continue to appear, of course, but often several days, a week, maybe two, after the show has opened. As a result, the more immediate means of information dissemination such as word of mouth, email and *sms* have become correspondingly more important. TV and radio do not brook deep discussions. They are about chat, not analysis. It takes very few TV and radio interview to teach you that, if you want to go on being invited onto these shows, you have to learn not to answer questions in any depth, but to bone up a few pat answers, and keep the jokes coming. The exceptions to this are rare.

Even when the arts do grab a bit of broad-reach space, what critics have to say is for the most part uninteresting, and frequently both ignorant and arrogant. (These last two epithets are well-known bedfellows.) Art is a three-legged stool—the artist (and product), the audience and the critical discourse surrounding the art. Weaken any one of these legs and the stool falls over. I think our stool is looking decidedly wobbly at the critical leg. I read review after review of the 'They-did-this-and-that-and-I-didn't-like-it' variety and then I re-read Maurice Berger, and realise again that most of our print-media critics—plus those in the popular electronic media—are at total odds with the conventional role of the critic:

> It is the critic, conventionally, who often supports or analyzes culture against the grain of popular tastes, indifference or hostility. In the best of circumstances, the critic serves as a kind of aesthetic mentor, introducing an audience to

> challenging, little-known, or obscure works, or offering insights that might make a work more accessible, engaging, profound, or relevant.[11]

This is the portrait of someone willing to debunk the myth of the mainstream. When I think of arts journalists and critics who make a livelihood out of confirming popular taste (and am told that to dislike certain things is to be 'un-Australian') of betraying sickening indifference towards the new and untried (measure it in the paltry column inches or minutes of airtime they give it) and, in many cases, of showing open hostility to anything beyond their very limited ken, I am angry at their flagrant abrogation of these responsibilities. We should not be amazed that those outside major arts or commercial organisations feel as if they are on their own. Their natural champion in that 'best of circumstances' has abandoned them to serve the myth of the mainstream.

We can't blame journalists for wanting to feed their families. If the owner wants this kind of medium, he will employ the kind of editor who will demand this kind of approach to the arts. But where are the arts editors who are fighting for something better? We have two, in Keith Gallasch and Virginia Baxter, at *RealTime*, which offers real analysis and champions the new, and we have them here and there in critics who do travel and at least glimpse the wide world of the arts, who strive to overcome what Berger calls the lethargy which 'exemplifies one of criticism's gravest problems: its tendency towards insularity and provincialism'.[12] In this context I see these two tendencies as powerful reinforcers of 'mainstream values'.

Berger continues:

> Given these and other problems, how can serious criticism remain relevant or even desirable in a country [the USA] where soundbites pass for erudite commentary, attention spans wane, and passion for the written word is becoming increasingly rare? Criticism must strive to be as resonant as the art it interprets, but without being abstruse or condescending.[13]

I think of the mornings when, foolishly, I glance at some review by some writer utterly unqualified to be passing judgment on some eminent international artist. And I feel waves of shame as I imagine that artist picking up that same paper and reading the trash that has gone to print about their life's work. Should I clarify? You can't insist that everyone likes everything, and I willingly embrace the fact of different tastes. What I can and do object to are cultural commentators who have a very limited experience of the arts on a global scale, have not travelled recently and have little upon which to base their judgment except personal taste, which does not qualify them to be a critic. I regard it as a case of genuine human injustice that those who have put their life's work and genius into a project can be publicly judged by parochial ignorami. It is akin to having a court case, the outcome of which will affect your life and work, decided by a bogus judge or biased jury. And yet we witness it every day of our lives. Some commentators, who lead very safe lives and have a desire to boost the myth of a mainstream, in which they see themselves as important standard-bearers, do not think twice before publicly humiliating the fragile creative efforts of artists:

> The strongest criticism today—the kind that offers hope for the vitality and future of the discipline—is capable of engaging, guiding, directing and influencing culture, even stimulating new forms of practice and expression. The strongest criticism serves as a dynamic, *critical* force, rather than as an act of boosterism. The strongest criticism uses language and rhetoric not merely for descriptive or evaluative purposes, but as means of inspiration, provocation, emotional connection, and experimentation.
>
> The strongest criticism also helps the reader to move beyond the surface details of the cultural artifact. Art is neither value-free nor an independent source of values; to one extent or another, it always reflects the needs, politics, intellectual and aesthetic priorities, and tastes of the artist, the institutions that support and disseminate his or her work, and a social and cultural universe of which both are part. By connecting the artifact and its institutions to the bigger picture of culture and society, the critic can, in effect, help readers better to understand the process and implications of art, the importance and problems of its institutions, and their relevance to their lives.[14]

While it is not always the case with less frequently-published serials, and certainly not with *RealTime*, the failure of art criticism in the popular mass media to accept these responsibilities means that art has lost one of its most important defenders against the myth of mainstream taste. Sadly, it has also lost a great artform in itself.

I see many of my close colleagues trying to assuage my anger and disappointment by trying to convince me that newsprint criticism is really no more than wrapping for fish and chips. But I am inconsolable. I am old enough to think back on performances of twenty years ago—What is my evidence? Stills, perhaps, or programs, prompt copies, recordings—and the critical discourse that surrounded them. As a contributor to Berger's book emphasises:

> In the instance of $100+ million movies, criticism may not be the most important index, *but it remains a register of values and perhaps most importantly it serves the historical record and our responsibility to vet the culture of our time with our best ideas and thinking.*[15]

I don't imagine anything's going to change soon: the media are commercial propositions. If a large number of people have fallen for the myth of the mainstream, helped in its creation by the mass media, then it behoves the media to go on reinforcing certain values that accord with that myth. All you ever hope for is just one journalist, just one arts editor, who will fight the good fight. Unlikely, however, since what our society values most highly are the things that money can buy: to have more money than someone else, you must be employed. On it goes. So maybe all you can hope for is the recognition of failed responsibility and some small measure to remedy the gross imbalance. Anything would be welcome at this stage.

6
Signs of the times—and what to do about them

The upward inflection has become endemic. The surest indication of a lack of confidence spreads like a plague amongst our people. Despite the constant assertions of patriotism—sometimes spawning jingoism—the word 'un-Australian', which has become the mainstream's demon and the Prime Minister's pitch for claiming mateship as a core spiritual promise at the heart of some statement of mainstream values, despite all this pro-mainstream propaganda and the PM's most valiant efforts, the youth of our nation have adopted the perfect indicator of a lack of confidence and robust identity—the upward vocal inflection. And their parents are following suit. Is it too outrageous to suggest that, if we had become a republic in time for the 2000 Olympic Games and apologised to Aboriginal Australians for the mistakes of the former British dependency, we might have avoided this plague of upward inflections and maintained the calm, reconciled, downward inflection that brings our spoken utterances to such a confident conclusion?

It was the Melbourne playwright Raimondo Cortese who first alerted me to the change that Australian expression was undergoing. In 1999 I saw his early success *Features of Blown Youth* and thought, 'In ten years' time I won't understand my own language.' Cortese has an uncanny ear for the way Australians speak. Perhaps it's his early years in the relative isolation of Tasmania, together with his Italian family background, but surely something inspired him to listen as an outsider to the speech of his compatriots and to record it accurately. The broken, unfinished sentences of his often feckless characters are splattered with upward inflections. The characters themselves are ill-defined, not at all like the decisive portraits, the decisive characters of David Williamson, a generation earlier. Whether right- or left-wing, upper-class, lower- or indeterminate, Williamson's characters had something solid to say and were not afflicted with the upward inflection. I want to say that we were surer of ourselves in the 1970s. Cortese's characters, by comparison, wander the streets, or live in squats, or gather accidentally at a badly-designed corner of concrete in the suburbs, and talk at odds with each other as sentence after sentence misses the mark. Their language fails them, and they illustrate what Ningali Lawford's grandfather (jabbi) told her, 'You lose your language, you lose your culture.'

People whose language fails them are unable to communicate, especially the most important things, the complex things, and they grab at superficiality and platitude as substitutes for real language and real communication. The subtlety of language, which should be the most prized gift of humanity, is abandoned. As passengers leap at midnight from the good ship *Apostrophe* into the icy waters of misinformation, the wreckage they cling to is captained by talk-back radio jocks and newsprint 'opinion'-mongers. They pose as defenders of a democracy in which ordinary people are given their say. This all turns out to be a mirage on the horizon, another wild suburban rumour. They cling in hope, but, alas, the rescue boat steered by Don Watson—now, in my fantasy, looking a bit like George Clooney in *The Perfect Storm*—may be too far away.[16]

And if art fails them too, then the cycle will take a lot longer to turn than many of us want. I wish Peter Garrett could have gone on winning battles through song, rather than by joining a political party.[17] I wish that writers and painters could win environmental battles through their art. I wish that the voice against injustice done to genuine refugees and the voice against declaring war for the first time on a nation who had not attacked us could have risen up potently in song, poetry, theatre and dance, and prevented Australia's reputation from being sullied in the wider world. I travel a lot outside Australia. I speak to people. I know that the opinion of Australia has changed.

Our artists, together, do offer a real picture of what Australia is. Not a homogeneous picture, perhaps, nor one that offers comfortable solutions, but these artists do have the courage to ask difficult questions. The pictures, together with stories, ideas, historical analysis, future thinking and questions which come from the widest possible range of Australians, can reflect what we truly are. Just as a country may well get the government it deserves, perhaps its art too is appropriate to it. Current resources are directed to the art that reflects the idea of a mainstream. But that isn't the whole truth, and those artists we need, to give us the real picture in all its fullness and complexity, are struggling to be heard.

Conclusion

To summarise: the public has bought the myth of the mainstream, and at present its ethos pervades every part of our lives. The bulk of government funding goes to support those arts deemed to reflect mainstream views. The loss of dialectic and the ascendancy of dogma, and the lack of respect for intellect in the broad public domain, make it difficult for a debate to be heard in which the myth is challenged and attention drawn to the different ways we connect and the things we share as a community. The space that debate occupies is also the space where art occurs, and it should be no wonder that just now in Australia art feels fragile while entertainment flourishes. The question is: what to do about it?

I've given clues throughout this essay to things that can be done, small strategies here and there. Mapping more general paths of action is harder. On the other hand, if artists and companies were to commit themselves to more urgent work than entertainment, then perhaps people would start to think differently about the assumptions that are made about them, and how those assumptions drive a national agenda.

Mikos Theodorakis once said that the only resistance is to be human. Under brutish regimes, this makes sense, but unfortunately, in apparently civilised states being human always seems to entail greed, territorialism, racism, violence and indifference. Hyperbole doesn't help change the mood, so it would be foolish to suggest that we are governed by a junta. In our Australia perhaps it would be better to start by trying to be humane, in the knowledge that simply by being human we follow the human cycle of reform and stasis.

Things being what they are at present, we shall encounter many in the arts who, understandably, for the sake of their jobs and their families will be quietly complicit with the prevailing attitudes. Every individual who refuses to comply will make a difference. Every artist who insists on being true to her or his art, every artist who insists on dealing, perhaps unfashionably, with urgent issues, every company that champions the new and the original, every philanthropist, corporation or politician who demands the same level of support be given to the classical canon and the unknown new work and forms. All these people will make a difference. Currency House is making a difference by publishing this new series of *Platform Papers*.

Subversion is a useful strategy: start with the known and familiar, draw people in, then introduce them, let them encounter the unknown and foreign, both in content and aesthetic. Bertolt Brecht wrote characters who were bad, but had good things about them, and good ones who had a mean streak. Things are never black and white: being a human being means living a lifetime of struggle, an ongoing dialectic. We must challenge the myth of the mainstream, which is said not to trust so many of us. Often it's merely a case of being aware, admitting it to ourselves, and challenging our own complicity, our own acceptance of the myth. Once a challenge is mounted internally on the root cause, ideas, works and actions bring that challenge out into the public arena.

I'm convinced there are already a good many people who don't believe in the myth of the mainstream—not just disgruntled lefties, but many so-called ordinary Australians, and new generations that include a breed of young corporates, for instance, who see through the marketing hype and could bring a fierce new energy to the support of new ideas. *In Conversation* with me at the recent Melbourne Festival, the great Canadian theatre-maker Robert Lepage described a Las Vegas that is full of such people right now. My advice is to take nothing for granted. If we in the arts community don't question the myth among ourselves, how can we find new ways and make new work that will challenge it in the broader community? And if the myth goes unchallenged, the spirit of art will continue to be marginalised. Those who believe we can afford that loss in the morass of mistakes and short-term thinking that make life on this earth increasingly pleasurable for the few and increasingly tortured for the many, those people need the power of art far more than they know.

Endnotes

1 John Howard's Coalition government was re-elected on 9 October 2004, as this essay was in gestation.
2 Tasmania's Festival of the Arts, of which I am currently advisor to the Artistic Program.
3 On 2 November 2004 American President George W. Bush was re-elected for a second term.
4 Casey Donovan was voted Australian Idol of 2004. Anthony Callea was runner-up.
5 Guy Sebastian, the first Australian Idol in 2003, is a product of the Paradise Community Church in the foothills of Adelaide.
6 During last year's federal election campaign Treasurer Costello urged an increase in population.
7 *Survival of the Fittest: the Artist versus the Corporate World*, *Platform Papers* 2 (Sydney: Currency House, 2004).
8 *Material Thinking: the Theory and Practice of Creative Research* (Carlton, Vic.: Melbourne University Press, 2004).
9 The Report of the government-instigated (Helen) Nugent Inquiry into major Australian arts organisations was handed down in July 1999.
10 The first, all-Australian *Ring* cycle—there was an imported one in 1913—played at Adelaide's Festival Theatre from 16 to 22 November 2004. Lisa Gasteen sang Brünnhilde. The production, with 97 opera

singers and 129 orchestral musicians, cost more than $15 million. I don't know the name of the Wagner fanatic from Los Angeles!

11 'Introduction: The Crisis of Criticism', in *The Crisis of Criticism*, ed. by Maurice Berger (New York: The New Press, 1998), p. 8.

12 Berger, p. 12.

13 Berger, p. 10.

14 Berger, p. 11.

15 In Berger, p. 156.

16 Don Watson is the author of *Death Sentence* (2003), on the infiltration of 'managerial language' into politics and *Watson's Dictionary of Weasel Words, Contemporary Cliché, Cant and Management Jargon* (2004), which speaks for itself.

17 At the recent 2004 federal election the former lead singer of Midnight Oil won the seat of Kingsford Smith for the Labor party.

Readers' Forum

Peter Eckersall on Platform Papers 3: *Trapped by the Past*

Julian Meyrick's insightful and urgent call for a deeper consideration of history, memory and intergenerational communication among contemporary theatre-makers is timely. His argument certainly rings true for the generation that tried to find work in theatre in the 1980s: in an era of declining funding the doors of the cultural sector were closed. Those who were fortunate enough to have work hung on to their jobs for the next ten (or twenty) years. Meanwhile, Meyrick, like many of us, started his own company—not a bad thing. But, as his analysis of MITP makes clear, creative output was never a problem; rather the lack of resources and financial support was, and continues to be, the burden of the independent arts.

Meyrick notes the decline in theatre production overall and the associated closure of medium-sized companies, a familiar if sobering story for artists and audiences. It is a strange anomaly that, while the populations of the main cities have increased dramatically over the last twenty years, the training of artists, the diversity of artistic production and the options for audiences have decreased almost to the same proportion. One is reminded of the proliferation of global flows amidst the decline of diversity and choice. As I will argue presently, in the double-speak of neo-liberal capitalism, in reality more is less.

Meyrick points to conflicts between old-school 'Anglo' and 1960s-generation New Wave theatre-makers in an effort to, in part, account for the fact of a shrinking repertoire. Aware that I may be oversimplifying the issues here, I shall call this a struggle between old and new left notions of culture and associated debates about the nature of cultural production. Certainly, a *Ganglands*-style critique of the cultural production of the baby-boomer generation is valid. The vision among baby-boomers of an Australian theatre has been criticised for being literal and bureaucratic, and 1980s and 1990s 'gatekeepers' were particularly active. However, while the generational split was intense, the notion that it prevented theatrical renewal perhaps needs further consideration.

I argue that theatre no longer operates in relation to debates between the old and new left. However clearly Meyrick identifies a powerful historical paradigm, these forces themselves no longer exert the influence they once did. Instead, the dominating order of neo-liberal capitalism, 'culture wars' and intense social euphoria have become the principal contexts for theatres' development. Let us briefly consider these aspects.

As Meyrick's essay demonstrates, regardless of the quality, theatre will be condemned by box-office failure. Inversely, conservative programming, and cute marketing will most probably signal success, if economic indicators are narrowly applied. The problem here is that a risk-adverse or excessively corporatist mindset is not good for theatre.

The second and third points speak more widely to the constraints of neo-liberal ideology and their impact on the arts. During the Howard years, social debate and cultural discourse in Australia have been shaped by surveillance, self-censure and hostility to a radical imagination. As a result, practically every mainstream cultural organisation has been subjected to political interference and ideological re-programming. Nevertheless, at crucial times, events programmed by a diversity of organisations including museums, galleries and public broadcasters have worked to make their fields of artistic production critically relevant. It is interesting to observe how little mainstream theatre has been willing or able to speak to the social condition in these ways. While a diversity of views is a characteristic of the independent theatre sector, the major performing arts organisations appear to be increasingly homogenised. Moreover, this theatre seems to be absorbed by euphoric and superficial sensibilities. As a result, it operates as a kind of globalised cultural product: the latest import, the revival, the summer musical, a night out with the stars. In Zygmunt Bauman's terms, this might be a globalised place of artistic inertia: 'Everything may happen but nothing can be done.' This kind of artistic levelling does not compare well with recent work by companies such as Not Yet It's Difficult (Melbourne), Performance Space (Sydney), Marrugeku (Sydney–based, but national), or the aforementioned major organisations in other fields of artistic production.

Seen in this light, Meyrick's argument seems to reach an endgame. On the one hand, new Australian plays have failed to attract audiences; on the other, so-called flagship companies are unable to develop new artistic forms. In responding to Meyrick's essay, then, we might add to the list of correctives a greater expectation that the whole community of Australian theatre turn its attention to issues of vital national importance and address them from divergent and critical perspectives. Imagine if a major theatre company programmed a whole season of works inspired by the themes of war or compassion, for example. This is not a utopian suggestion; rather it acknowledges an historical function of art to give insight. Thus, we might come to expect a more radical political and aesthetic stance for theatre. Ironically, this lynchpin united the two former generations of theatre-makers who, despite their differences, were deeply committed to the idea that theatre was a form of social construction and cultural intervention.

Meyrick's essay points to the fact that structural and cultural issues are interrelated. Theatre should be a cultural project of national importance. His argument is cogent and well worth making. We shall wait with interest to see whether, when, and how the fruits of his labour impress upon the major companies.

Chris Mead on the plight of the playwright:

About this time last year two leading female playwrights established a writers' group. The propitious moment of its founding was beleaguered, however, by total doubt. What were they, a trauma support group or crucible for ideas? With so few opportunities for playwrights one of the writers wondered whether they should actually just give up writing for the theatre altogether. Maybe, she pondered aloud, only five people Australia-wide should be allowed to be playwrights at any one time. Maybe, she continued, since there was a living to be made by only a handful of theatre writers, everyone else should just retire. And this was not simply sour grapes or bitter anecdotage, but the ugly end of theatre pragmatism. An alarming moment indeed.

Julian Meyrick's paper rings similar alarm bells. Containing, as it does, provocation, allegation, fact and insult, it is a familiar trope—the call to arms. Every few years—or maybe perhaps only at moments of generational friction and change—the sky falls in. This is a good and necessary hue and cry, for Meyrick has re-activated the mechanism at the heart of theatre history—it is always dying, always in crisis, always needing adversity/enmity/imminent destruction to revive, thrive and survive. His argument is cogent and meaty and difficult to refute (once one realises his terms of reference). And things now are worse than ever before. For sure. What was most startling about Meyrick's argument is the way in which it has been interpreted by his readers, including the press.

Sure, there are loads of plays as well as playwrights by the lorry load, and, sure, it feels a little bit like there's a boom in theatre at the moment—OK, maybe just a resurgence, and look, Ma, with almost no cash!—but, so what? Meyrick asks in no uncertain terms why theatre's intellectual substructure is so bereft. We barely look back at all, and certainly not in anger; the serious damage was done years ago, but we've given up trying to fix it, happy to make do and improvise with the exigencies. As a result, the middle has been punched out of the industry. And we respond by saying (a) it's not about the generation gap, 'cos we all get along just fine, cough, cough; (b) I wuz robbed; (c) the glass is half full (tours, Urban Theatre Projects, pumping Fringe etc.); (d) but things would probably be better if we had more money; and (e) he's Melbourne-centric, and did I mention tours and UTP? Intellectual substructure? Infrastructure reform? Err, well, no, probably not.

Meyrick suggests that there is a deep structural malaise here that has gone unacknowledged, the legacy of an ad hoc industry. And a reactive industry lacks genuine vision, most especially with respect to new writing. Where is, for instance, a Granville Barker, Devine, or Daldry to kickstart new work with the resources it needs? Can't blame the audience. Maybe it's the population size? Unlikely. Development has been divorced from production, fringe from mainstream, boomer from X. Gaps and lacunae are the order of the day. Where is the middle ground, i.e. the 'small-to-medium' theatres that generate new work? What are we going to do about it? What's the point of a fancy smokestack if there's no coal and the engine's on the fritz?

I asked a similar question at last year's National Playwrights' Conference in a session I had pretentiously called 'Colloquy'. The response was something like 'enough already'. The gathered professional folk didn't want to sit around gasbagging any more about our woes. Instead, they wanted to get on and do it, move plays closer to production, get actors moving, writers writing and audiences laughing, thinking, feeling. Just do it. Sure. And the vision thing? The middle ground? Well, maybe, next year.

John McCallum on Playbox's honourable repertoire:

Julian Meyrick's essay has many provocative things to say about the state of our theatre, but one thing he does not comment upon, and that hasn't been mentioned in the press coverage since the essay appeared, is Playbox Theatre's actual repertoire. A central plank of his argument is based on a simple quantitative table of box-office data entitled 'Paid Attendances at Playbox Theatre, 1998–2003' (pp. 67–9). This was picked up in a feature in the *Age* by Robin Usher with the heading 'Getting Bums on Seats' (1 February 2005). The table is used to argue that the funding for Playbox to do new work hasn't been as effective as it should have been, that there is now no 'middle ground' of small-to-medium companies with the resources to develop new work and that the old guard of the New Wave generation has failed to hand on the baton to new young artists.

I am based in Sydney and have no axe to grind about the politics of Melbourne theatre, but there are obviously two ways of looking at this table. One is to observe the poor attendance figures, including the clear decline over the five years, which Meyrick notes. The other is to look qualitatively at the plays they did. The Playbox repertoire, even if we only take the five years covered in Meyrick's table, is impressive. More importantly, in the light of his argument, it clearly straddles the generations. Many of the plays have had a national impact, and all of them have been published. This is part of Playbox's legacy.

Usher quoted the public funding figures for Playbox ($1.374 million a year) and the MTC ($1.574 million a year), and commented that MTC had used not much more money to present a longer, more varied season. Well, duh. MTC doesn't need as much money, pro rata, because it has a large established audience base—the audience that Michael Kantor says he now wants to attract to Malthouse. It costs money to do what Playbox has been doing, producing between eight and 14 new plays each year. Naturally, there is a significant failure rate. Maybe there are selection issues. The fact that audiences don't always come to new Australian work is well-known—ask anyone in the film industry. The two off-the-graph box-office hits of the five years of Meyrick's data were Black Swan's and Belvoir's visiting production *Cloudstreet* and *Secret Bridesmaids' Business*, a cheerful but inconsequential commercial play. But if you want to add concerns about the value of the arts to a bums-on-seats measure of success then look at the rest of the repertoire. Here are a few examples from the five years of the table, using Meyrick's data.

In 1998 Andrew Bovell's *Speaking in Tongues* played to 74% capacity—not bad, but it had an even larger audience when it was made into the film *Lantana*. In 1999 *Cloudstreet* reached 93%—not surprisingly—but Louis Nowra's great Asian historical drama *The Language of the Gods* only made 29%. In 2000 David Williamson's *Face to Face*, admittedly one of his best plays of the last ten years, played to 80%, while Michael Gurr's interesting *Crazy Brave* and Debra Oswald's fine underdog drama *Sweet Road* only played to 28% and 47% respectively.

In 2001 one of Melbourne and Australia's most distinguished New Wave playwrights, John Romeril, had his adventurous *Miss Tanaka* (57%), and the young urban writer Raimondo Cortese had his provocative *St Kilda Tales* (51%). In the same year one of the most important and powerful plays ever written about Australia's dark heritage, Andrew Bovell's *Holy Day*, played to 34%; and Dorothy Hewett's last play, *Nowhere*, a wonderful distillation of a lot of what she had been trying to say throughout her career, played to 58%—again, not too bad, but less than you'd expect for one of the greatest writers for the stage of the last 50 years.

In 2002 there was an important season of studio productions of new plays by black Australians, including Richard J. Frankland's *Conversations With the Dead* (okay, it was more of a success in Neil Armfield's later Belvoir production, but it was Playbox that made it happen) and the premiere of Daniel Keene's astonishingly beautiful, theatrically eloquent, multi-award-winning play, *Half and Half*, and also of Joanna Murray-Smith's successful *Rapture*. In 2003 Playbox commissioned and produced Stephen Sewell's *Myth, Propaganda and Disaster in Nazi Germany and Contemporary America*. At the time of writing, it is in its third Australian production and about to be produced in New York and London. That year there was also Ben Ellis's astonishing anti-New Wave play *Falling Petals,* and Matt Cameron's magic fable of the dark side of suburban life, *Ruby Moon*. Whatever you think of these plays—and, obviously, I've picked the ones I admire—you cannot say that Playbox's repertoire has been insignificant. And you can't say that bums-on-seats are a measure of value.

I worry that the debate provoked by Meyrick's essay will throw up a model in which the new work of adventurous young artists will be seen merely as grist for the mainstream mill. New writers need to have their work produced, not endlessly workshopped, and Playbox at least did that. (And this year Griffin, Malthouse and Black Swan are all making their spaces available to smaller companies that actually do shows as well as productions.) I hate to sound like an old New Waver, but let's not pretend that 'paid attendances' are the only measure.

On Thursday 20 January 2005, at the Stables Theatre, in Sydney, a public discussion/forum was held on the subject of Julian Meyrick's Platform Paper. Julian Meyrick's opening statement was followed by contributions by Rob Brookman, Lyn Wallis and David Berthold.

Lyn Wallis addresses the Next Wave:

Julian's Meyrick's essay, *Why our Theatre is Facing Paralysis*, raises many fascinating questions about the links between generations of artists.

I am one of the last wave of theatre-makers to have enjoyed the nurturing support of a particular segment of Meyrick's 'middle ground', before it crumbled in the wake of 'mainstream-to-the-regions' touring initiatives such as Playing Australia. For me and other artists of my age, this 'middle ground' was represented by regional and community theatre companies. When the death knell sounded for many of these, another valuable commodity was lost, a vital *training ground* for artists at entry level. In terms of an organic system of development and mentorship through intergenerational contact, nothing has really replaced it. Twenty years on, I find myself working as a mentor and facilitator with the Next Wave. Together with dynamic independent companies being primped and preened by 'season hubs' such as B Sharp and its brothers- and sisters-in-arms across the country, this Next Wave of artists and producers is staging a little cultural tsunami all of its own.

There has been no 'middle ground' for them and, in response to being exiled, they've grabbed some tools from the family shed and determinedly dug a corner patch in some bloody hard soil. I strongly suspect that *this* wave is a lot like the *old* New Wave; they are a rambunctious, confident and slightly anarchic lot, who certainly aren't thinking about what they are creating in a cohesive way at all, but are responding purely out of *need* and out of an instinct that tells them what's missing in the general scene. Working collectively in a very fluid way, they are addressing some of our past mistakes. We should pay their efforts some serious attention.

First, they are actively bridging the divide between artists and facilitators. It's a joy to have joint meetings with Next Wave directors and producers, in which conversations about art, money and audiences overlap and intertwine, in which there are mutual admiration and support, and a recognition that each one of us would have a much more difficult time of it without the others.

Secondly, the Next Wave is not altogether abandoning its patch of soil when more lucrative opportunities come along. There is an investment going on here which is not just about using the fringe as a stepping stone, or as a place to work when there is no other work, but as a place to work willfully, to engage with one's peers in a passionate endeavour, to create a kind of theatre that may not be happening elsewhere and, sometimes, to do *great* work. How is this wave of indie artists hanging in there, albeit by their fingernails? The creation of 'season hubs' has certainly helped. Sydney is at the forefront of this trend, but examples of it are to be found in most states and territories.

So, is this relatively new territory, *solid* ground? No, it isn't. I am fearful, because I see this fantastic bit of turf erupting before my eyes, and yet in my heart I know it could just be like Brigadoon, a beautiful, unreal place that only appears for one day every hundred years. The reality is that most of these artists, producers and technicians are working for next to nothing and that, if they didn't pour their blood, sweat and tears onto those little patches of earth, we wouldn't have the jewel-like flower we have now—the liveliest, most cohesive, best independent scene we may *ever* have had. It desperately needs more resources, and quickly—before these groups grow weary of the penniless grind.

What about formal development strategies? At present, our most damaging practice is to identify the best and brightest and to propel them with all the force of a Saturn V rocket into the stratosphere. Yes, it's the 'Hot Young Thing Ballistic Arts Program'! Guaranteed to get your picture on television, but also to render you paralysed by motion-sickness and lofty heights! And then, of course, there's re-entry—without a heat-shield. But, surely, we are helping here? No, it isn't help, it isn't development and, in truth, it's rarely survivable. As we jump up and down in our desperation and good-hearted enthusiasm to get the future on the road, we better make damn sure we're not trampling our prodigies to death in the process. Beautiful gardens take time to grow. And this new patch of ground has enormous potential—but it will only flourish with help, and a more considered approach to its development.

Nicholas Pickard responds to David Berthold's contribution to the Stables forum, from which an edited extract was published in the *Australian* on 27 January 2005.

In responding to Julian Meyrick's argument, David Berthold asks, 'Have any of these [professional theatre] companies, over the past decade, taken up an inspired independent production and worked to develop it?' But Berthold makes no mention of the efforts of the fringe scene outside of the independent theatre scene. I refer to the fringe as a body of practitioners who exist without the support or approval of an independent venue. They are the theatre practitioners that can't get past a submission process, let alone break into paid work at a flagship theatre company.

My experience is a case in point. While completing my postgraduate directing studies at the Academy of Theatre, University of Ljubljana in Slovenia, I commissioned an Australian playwright to write a play for six actors, all graduating students. As we received the script in stages by email from Sydney, we spent an exciting three months workshopping, rehearsing and re-writing in an atmosphere of cultural exchange and bi-lingual confusion.The result was a critically-acclaimed production that has been seen by audiences from the far-reaches of the Balkans and throughout central Europe. One of the most interesting reactions came from a Slovenian reviewer: 'It is possible to recognise distinguishable features of modern time and space in a story from such a far-off continent. To the audience the story seems extremely close, happening at our end of the global village, so to speak.' Our cross-cultural collaboration had worked: we had created theatre that was new, unique and 'universal'.

It is interesting to compare this show's success at several European festivals, to the lukewarm reception it received in Australia. After three years and ten submissions we have given up trying to remount the show here, and have resorted to more 'commercial' submissions that seem more likely to gain the attention of independent-theatre decision- makers. The real disappointment for me, however, has been that approaching independent theatres with proposals based on development and collaboration has received only negative reactions. But my principal concern is the lack of variety in our independent theatre-work, particularly new Australian playwriting that puts our directors, designers and actors to the test, that is inherently theatrical and seeks to develop the craft of theatre, that is risk-taking and unique to Australia.

A major problem with the independent scene in Sydney is the effect of the current submission process. The criteria for success are weighted almost entirely towards the commercial/marketing/advertorial merits of a project. Each venue receives over 100 competing submissions each year, thus diluting much of what practitioners want to do—the effect is catastrophic. The result for independent theatre and its audiences is that these 60–100-seat venues, all desperate to stay commercially viable, make conservative and predictable programming decisions. Exciting and challenging theatre is pushed aside, uneconomic and irrelevant.

The inspiration I derive from people in Sydney's theatre scene to create exciting theatre, new scripts, new ideas, and their willingness to experiment, often without financial or other support, is a constant source of encouragement. The balance, however, between inspired theatre and the lightweight, thematically conservative fare currently on our stages needs to be adjusted: what we need is theatre that, by means of a range of investigative processes and collaborative rehearsal, tries to break down boundaries between scripted theatre, physical theatre and performance art.

I don't pretend to know how independent theatres should be run, but I believe that the most effective way of forcing professional theatre to take up 'inspired independent productions' is to actively encourage its creation. I believe that audiences are yearning for originality, and if independent theatre can provide it, professional commercial theatre-makers will be obliged to rethink their programs and practices. For all of us, to coin a phrase, it's probably a case of who dares will win.

Contributors

Dr Peter Eckersall

Dr Peter Eckersall, who teaches at the University of Melbourne, researches in the fields of Japanese theatre, theatre and society, and dramaturgy. Co-founder of The Men Who Knew Too Much and currently resident dramaturg of Not Yet It's Difficult, he has recently edited *Alternatives: Debating Theatre Culture in an Age of Confusion* (2004), essays on inter-culturalism, theatre, and globalisation.

Chris Mead

Chris Mead is the Curator of the Australian National Playwrights Conference and Festival Director of World Interplay, the International Festival for Young Playwrights. His PhD, in Australian History, was awarded by Sydney University and he was Literary Manager of Company B Belvoir between 2000 and 2003.

John McCallum

John McCallum is the *Australian*'s Sydney theatre critic, a lecturer at the University of NSW and Acting Chair of the Australian National Playwrights' Centre.

Lyn Wallis

Lyn Wallis has worked as a director, performer and teacher for over twenty years. As Downstairs Theatre Director for Sydney's Company B Belvoir, she has just programmed her seventh B Sharp season.

Nicholas Pickard

Nicholas Pickard is a Sydney-based theatre director. His contact details are: nickpickard@hotmail.com, ph 0412 212 291